Introduction

Welcome to the world of holistic blood sugar mastery. In these pages, we embark on a transformative journey inspired by the holistic philosophy of Dr. Sebi, a visionary thinker whose principles guide us toward optimal well-being.

As you begin this exploration, it's essential to recognize that the path to balanced blood sugar levels and vibrant health is not a one-size-fits-all solution. Instead, it's a holistic approach that encompasses every aspect of your life. It's a journey of self-discovery, empowerment, and vitality.

This book is a roadmap, a guide to help you navigate this path to holistic blood sugar control. It's a culmination of Dr. Sebi's wisdom and principles, translated into practical steps that you can incorporate into your daily life. Whether you're seeking to prevent blood sugar imbalances, manage diabetes, or simply optimize your health, the holistic approach is a foundation for lifelong well-being.

In the chapters that follow, we'll delve deep into the principles of Dr. Sebi's philosophy, exploring the significance of an alkaline-rich diet, the power of herbal remedies, the importance of mindful eating, the role of physical activity, the healing potential of sleep, stress reduction, proper hydration, and the transformative power of detoxification.

Each chapter is a building block, offering insights, strategies, and practical steps to empower you on your holistic blood sugar journey. Whether you're new to holistic health or well-versed in its principles, there's something here for everyone. We'll guide you through the science, the practices, and the mindset needed to achieve and maintain stable blood sugar levels.

As you read, remember that this journey is uniquely yours. What works for one person may not work exactly the same for another. Embrace the flexibility and adaptability of the holistic approach. Listen to your body, trust your intuition, and be patient with yourself as you navigate this path.

At the heart of this journey is the understanding that you have the power to shape your health and future. You are the steward of your body and mind, and your choices today have a profound impact on your well-being and the well-being of generations to come.

So, let's begin this journey together. Let's explore the holistic principles that can help you achieve blood sugar mastery and vibrant health. Whether you're taking your first step or continuing your path, know that you have the knowledge, tools, and inner strength to master your holistic blood sugar journey.

As you turn each page, may you uncover inspiration, wisdom, and the empowerment to embrace a future filled with vitality and joy.

Welcome to your journey of holistic blood sugar mastery.

Table of Contents

Chapter 1: Dr. Sebi's Holistic Approach to Blood Sugar Control

In the world of holistic health, few names command as much respect and recognition as that of Dr. Sebi. Born Alfredo Darrington Bowman in 1933 in Honduras, Dr. Sebi dedicated his life to unlocking the secrets of nature to promote healing and vitality. His unique approach to health and wellness has touched the lives of countless individuals, offering hope and transformation, particularly in the realm of blood sugar control.

Understanding Dr. Sebi's Philosophy

Dr. Sebi's holistic philosophy revolves around the fundamental concept that the human body is an extraordinary, self-sustaining organism capable of healing itself when provided with the right conditions. At the heart of his teachings is the belief that nature, in its purest form, offers the key to health and longevity.

Dr. Sebi's philosophy encompasses several key principles:

Alkaline Diet: Dr. Sebi advocated for the consumption of an alkaline-based diet, rich in foods that support the body's natural alkalinity. He believed that an acidic diet, often characterized by processed foods, sugars, and meats, was at the root of many health problems, including elevated blood sugar levels.

Bioelectric Cell Food: Dr. Sebi emphasized the importance of consuming foods with a high bioelectric cell content. These are foods that resonate at the same frequency as our body's cells, promoting cellular health and optimal function.

Herbal Remedies: Central to Dr. Sebi's philosophy were the healing properties of herbs. He believed that specific herbs possessed the ability to cleanse and revitalize the body, ultimately helping to balance blood sugar and promote overall well-being.

The Connection between Diet and Blood Sugar

One of the cornerstones of Dr. Sebi's teachings is the profound impact of diet on blood sugar levels. He contended that many of the modern health challenges we face, including diabetes and high blood sugar, stem from dietary choices that disrupt the body's natural equilibrium.

Dr. Sebi's approach to blood sugar control can be summarized in these key points:

Eliminating Acidic Foods: Dr. Sebi advocated for the removal of acidic foods, such as processed sugars, artificial additives, and heavily processed meats, from the diet. These foods are believed to contribute to blood sugar imbalances.

Embracing Alkaline Foods: Central to Dr. Sebi's dietary recommendations were alkaline foods like leafy greens, fruits, and nuts. These foods promote an alkaline environment in the body, which is conducive to stable blood sugar levels.

Herbal Support: Dr. Sebi often prescribed specific herbs known for their blood sugar-regulating properties, such as bitter melon and burdock root. These herbs were believed to assist the body in maintaining healthy glucose levels.

Dr. Sebi's holistic approach to blood sugar control provides an alternative perspective on managing this critical aspect of health. By understanding his philosophy and embracing his principles, individuals seeking to reduce blood sugar levels can embark on a journey toward better well-being, one rooted in the wisdom of nature.

In the chapters that follow, we will delve deeper into Dr. Sebi's teachings, exploring specific dietary recommendations, the role of herbs in blood sugar control, and practical steps to implement his holistic approach in your life. By the end of this journey, you'll have the knowledge and tools to embark on your path to holistic blood sugar control, the Dr. Sebi way.

<u>**Chapter 2: Alkaline Foods for Blood Sugar Balance**</u>

In our journey to unlock the secrets of blood sugar control through Dr. Sebi's holistic approach, we arrive at a cornerstone of his philosophy: the profound impact of alkaline foods. Dr. Sebi believed that by embracing an alkaline-rich diet, we can create an internal environment that supports stable blood sugar levels and overall health.

Exploring Alkaline-Rich Foods

Dr. Sebi's dietary recommendations revolve around the consumption of foods that promote an alkaline environment in the body. These foods, often referred to as "alkaline foods," are characterized by their ability to balance the body's pH levels and create an environment conducive to optimal health and blood sugar regulation.

Key alkaline-rich foods include:

<u>Leafy Greens:</u> Spinach, kale, collard greens, and Swiss chard are examples of leafy greens that top Dr. Sebi's list. They are not only packed with essential nutrients but are also highly alkaline.

<u>Fresh Fruits:</u> Many fruits, such as berries, melons, and apples, are naturally alkaline. They provide a wealth of vitamins, minerals, and fiber while supporting blood sugar balance.

<u>Nuts and Seeds:</u> Almonds, pumpkin seeds, and chia seeds are excellent sources of alkaline-forming foods. They offer healthy fats, protein, and essential minerals.

<u>Herbs:</u> Dr. Sebi frequently incorporated herbs into his dietary recommendations due to their alkalizing properties. Herbs like dandelion, chamomile, and elderberry were often utilized for their health benefits.

How Alkaline Foods Support Blood Sugar Balance

The consumption of alkaline foods aligns with Dr. Sebi's philosophy of promoting an internal environment that fosters blood sugar stability. Here's how alkaline foods contribute to this balance:

<u>Regulating pH Levels:</u> Alkaline foods help maintain a slightly alkaline pH level in the body, which is believed to support stable blood sugar levels.

<u>Nutrient Density:</u> Alkaline-rich foods are typically packed with essential nutrients like vitamins, minerals, and antioxidants. These nutrients play a role in regulating blood sugar and promoting overall health.

<u>Fiber Content:</u> Many alkaline foods are high in dietary fiber. Fiber slows the absorption of glucose in the bloodstream, preventing rapid spikes in blood sugar levels after meals.

<u>Reducing Inflammatory Load:</u> Alkaline foods are often anti-inflammatory in nature. Chronic inflammation can contribute to insulin resistance and elevated blood sugar, making anti-inflammatory foods crucial for blood sugar control.

Incorporating Alkaline Foods into Your Diet

Now that we've explored the significance of alkaline foods in Dr. Sebi's approach, let's discuss practical steps for incorporating these foods into your diet:

Start with Leafy Greens: Incorporate leafy greens like spinach and kale into your daily meals. They make excellent additions to salads, smoothies, and cooked dishes.

Enjoy Fresh Fruits: Opt for fresh fruits as snacks or desserts. Berries, apples, and citrus fruits are not only delicious but also alkaline-rich.

Nuts and Seeds as Snacks: Almonds, pumpkin seeds, and chia seeds can be consumed as snacks or added to your breakfast or yogurt.

Explore Alkaline Herbs: Consider incorporating alkaline herbs like dandelion or chamomile into your herbal teas or as seasonings in your cooking.

By gradually introducing these alkaline foods into your diet, you can create a balanced and health-supportive approach to blood sugar control. In the next chapters, we'll delve deeper into Dr. Sebi's holistic principles, including the role of herbal remedies and fasting, as we continue our journey towards mastering blood sugar control the Dr. Sebi way.

Chapter 3: The Importance of Herbal Remedies

In our exploration of Dr. Sebi's holistic approach to blood sugar control, we venture into a realm that held immense significance in his philosophy: the utilization of herbal remedies. Dr. Sebi firmly believed that specific herbs possessed the natural power to cleanse, rejuvenate, and support the body in maintaining healthy blood sugar levels.

Dr. Sebi's Advocacy for Herbal Healing

Dr. Sebi's reverence for the natural world extended to the belief that herbs, as gifts from nature, harbored remarkable healing properties. He often referred to herbs as the keys to unlocking the body's innate ability to heal and achieve optimal health.

Key principles guiding Dr. Sebi's approach to herbal remedies:

Herbs as Balancing Agents: Dr. Sebi viewed herbs as natural balancers, capable of harmonizing the body's internal systems, including blood sugar regulation.

Herbs for Cellular Cleansing: He believed that herbs had the capacity to detoxify cells, removing accumulated waste and toxins that could disrupt blood sugar balance.

Herbs for Nourishment: Certain herbs, in Dr. Sebi's philosophy, provided vital nutrients and trace elements that supported overall health and blood sugar control.

Specific Herbs for Blood Sugar Control

Dr. Sebi had a selection of favored herbs renowned for their potential to assist in blood sugar regulation:

Bitter Melon (Momordica charantia): Bitter melon is a well-known herb often recommended for its potential to lower blood sugar levels. It contains compounds that may improve insulin sensitivity.

Burdock Root (Arctium lappa): Burdock root is esteemed for its blood-purifying properties. It is believed to assist in detoxifying the bloodstream and promoting healthy blood sugar levels.

Cinnamon (Cinnamomum verum): Cinnamon is a versatile herb and spice that may help improve insulin sensitivity and reduce insulin resistance.

Fenugreek (Trigonella foenum-graecum): Fenugreek seeds have shown promise in several studies for their potential to lower blood sugar levels and improve glycemic control.

Incorporating Herbal Remedies into Your Routine

If you're interested in incorporating herbal remedies into your blood sugar management plan, it's essential to do so with care and understanding. Here are some steps to consider:

Consultation: Before starting any herbal regimen, it's wise to consult with a healthcare professional or herbalist who can provide guidance tailored to your specific needs and circumstances.

Research: Educate yourself about the herbs you plan to use. Understand their potential benefits, recommended dosages, and any possible interactions with medications.

Quality Matters: Ensure that you source high-quality herbs from reputable suppliers. Organic, sustainably sourced herbs are often preferred.

<u>Consistency:</u> Consistency is key when using herbal remedies. Follow recommended dosages and give your body time to respond to the herbs' effects.

<u>Monitor Progress:</u> Keep track of your blood sugar levels as you incorporate herbal remedies. This will help you gauge their effectiveness and make any necessary adjustments to your regimen.

Dr. Sebi's reverence for the natural world and his belief in the healing power of herbs continue to inspire individuals seeking holistic approaches to blood sugar control. As we journey through this book, we'll further explore Dr. Sebi's holistic principles, including the role of fasting and mindful eating, to help you achieve optimal blood sugar balance and overall well-being.

Chapter 4: Fasting and Intermittent Fasting in Dr. Sebi's World

In our quest to uncover the holistic secrets of blood sugar control according to Dr. Sebi's philosophy, we arrive at a transformative concept: fasting. Dr. Sebi recognized fasting, in its various forms, as a powerful tool that aligns with his principles of natural healing and blood sugar management.

How Fasting Aligns with Dr. Sebi's Philosophy

Dr. Sebi's holistic approach emphasizes the body's innate ability to heal itself when provided with the right conditions. Fasting, he believed, created an environment within the body conducive to healing and balance. Here's how fasting aligns with Dr. Sebi's philosophy:

Rest and Repair: Fasting offers the digestive system a rest, redirecting the body's energy towards repair and rejuvenation. This can be especially beneficial for individuals seeking to improve blood sugar regulation.

Detoxification: Dr. Sebi often referred to fasting as a natural detoxification process. By abstaining from solid food for a defined period, the body has an opportunity to eliminate accumulated toxins that might contribute to blood sugar imbalances.

Cellular Health: Fasting can support the health of individual cells. When the body is in a fasting state, cells may become more sensitive to insulin, which can enhance blood sugar control.

Exploring Fasting Techniques

Dr. Sebi advocated for various fasting techniques, each with its unique benefits. Here are some of the fasting approaches aligned with his philosophy:

Water Fasting: Water fasting involves abstaining from all foods and consuming only water for a designated period, typically ranging from 24 hours to several days. Dr. Sebi often recommended water fasting as a potent tool for detoxification and resetting the body's systems.

Juice Fasting: Juice fasting allows the consumption of freshly prepared fruit and vegetable juices while refraining from solid foods. This approach provides essential nutrients while still promoting detoxification and rest.

Intermittent Fasting: Intermittent fasting involves cycling between periods of eating and fasting. This approach can support blood sugar regulation by allowing the body to become more insulin-sensitive during fasting periods.

Fasting-Mimicking Diet: Dr. Sebi's philosophy aligns with the concept of a fasting-mimicking diet, which involves consuming very few calories and specific nutrients during a short-term fasting period, usually around five days. This approach offers some of the benefits of fasting while providing essential nutrients.

Incorporating Fasting Safely

While fasting can offer numerous benefits for blood sugar control and overall health, it's essential to approach it safely and mindfully. Here are some considerations when incorporating fasting into your lifestyle:

Consultation: Consult with a healthcare professional before embarking on any fasting regimen, especially if you have underlying health conditions or are taking medications.

Start Gradually: If you're new to fasting, consider starting with shorter fasts and gradually extending the duration as you become more accustomed to the process.

Stay Hydrated: Ensure you drink enough water or fluids during fasting periods to prevent dehydration.

Monitor Blood Sugar: If you have diabetes or other blood sugar-related conditions, closely monitor your blood sugar levels during fasting and consult with your healthcare provider for guidance.

Breaking the Fast: Be mindful of how you break your fast. Choose nourishing, easily digestible foods to reintroduce to your diet.

Fasting is a powerful tool in Dr. Sebi's holistic approach to blood sugar control. As we continue our journey through this book, we'll explore additional aspects of Dr. Sebi's philosophy, including the role of mindful eating and the importance of dietary choices in achieving optimal blood sugar balance.

As we delve deeper into Dr. Sebi's holistic approach to blood sugar control, we encounter a profound aspect of his philosophy: the significance of mindful eating and conscious dietary choices. Dr. Sebi believed that being present and intentional in our eating habits is essential for maintaining stable blood sugar levels and overall health.

The Significance of Mindful Eating

Mindful eating is a practice rooted in mindfulness, the art of being fully present in the moment. Dr. Sebi recognized its potential to transform our relationship with food and positively impact blood sugar control. Here's why mindful eating matters:

Awareness of Hunger and Fullness: Mindful eating encourages us to listen to our bodies, recognizing when we are genuinely hungry and when we are satisfied. This can help prevent overeating, which can lead to blood sugar spikes.

Savoring Food: By savoring each bite, we derive more pleasure from our meals. This satisfaction can reduce the need for excessive snacking and sugary treats.

Emotional Eating: Mindful eating helps us identify emotional triggers for eating, such as stress or boredom, allowing us to address these issues without turning to food.

Conscious Choices: It encourages making conscious dietary choices, selecting foods that align with Dr. Sebi's principles of an alkaline, herb-rich diet.

Practical Strategies for Mindful Eating

Dr. Sebi's holistic approach to blood sugar control encourages mindful eating as a fundamental practice. Here are some practical strategies to incorporate into your daily routine:

Eat Without Distractions: Avoid eating in front of the TV, computer, or while scrolling through your phone. Focus solely on your meal.

Chew Thoroughly: Chew each bite slowly and thoroughly. This aids digestion and allows your body to signal when you're full.

Engage Your Senses: Pay attention to the colors, textures, and flavors of your food. Engaging your senses enhances the dining experience.

Pause Between Bites: Put your utensils down between bites. This simple act encourages you to savor your food and prevents mindless eating.

Practice Gratitude: Take a moment before your meal to express gratitude for the nourishment it provides. This can foster a positive relationship with food.

Making Conscious Dietary Choices

In Dr. Sebi's philosophy, conscious dietary choices play a pivotal role in blood sugar management. These choices align with his principles of an alkaline, herb-rich diet. Here's how to make conscious dietary choices:

<u>Choose Alkaline Foods:</u> Prioritize alkaline-rich foods, such as leafy greens, fruits, and nuts. These foods support stable blood sugar levels.

<u>Incorporate Herbs:</u> Explore the use of herbs known for their blood sugar-regulating properties, such as bitter melon and burdock root.

<u>Avoid Processed Foods:</u> Steer clear of heavily processed and sugary foods. These can disrupt blood sugar balance.

<u>Read Labels:</u> Become a vigilant label reader. Look for hidden sugars and additives in packaged foods.

<u>Plan Meals:</u> Plan your meals in advance to ensure they align with Dr. Sebi's principles. This prevents impulsive, less healthful choices.

Mindful eating and conscious dietary choices are powerful tools in your journey towards blood sugar control. As we continue our exploration of Dr. Sebi's holistic approach, we'll delve into the significance of physical activity, herbal remedies, and other aspects of his philosophy to help you achieve optimal well-being.

Chapter 6: Physical Activity as a Natural Blood Sugar Regulator

In our ongoing exploration of Dr. Sebi's holistic approach to blood sugar control, we arrive at a fundamental aspect of his philosophy: the role of physical activity in maintaining stable blood sugar levels and overall well-being.

Dr. Sebi's Perspective on Exercise

Dr. Sebi held a perspective on physical activity that was firmly rooted in the belief that movement and exercise are essential components of a holistic, health-focused lifestyle. He recognized that a sedentary lifestyle could contribute to blood sugar imbalances and a range of health issues. Here's why physical activity matters in Dr. Sebi's philosophy:

Improved Insulin Sensitivity: Regular physical activity can enhance the body's sensitivity to insulin, the hormone responsible for regulating blood sugar. This can result in more effective blood sugar control.

Enhanced Glucose Uptake: Exercise promotes the uptake of glucose by muscles, reducing the amount of sugar circulating in the bloodstream.

Weight Management: Physical activity contributes to weight management, which is crucial for individuals with blood sugar concerns. Maintaining a healthy weight can help improve blood sugar regulation.

Stress Reduction: Dr. Sebi also recognized exercise as a means of reducing stress, which can have a positive impact on blood sugar levels.

Dr. Sebi's Recommendations for Physical Activity

While Dr. Sebi emphasized the importance of physical activity, he did not prescribe rigid exercise routines. Instead, he advocated for movement that aligns with an individual's preferences and lifestyle. Here are some key principles in Dr. Sebi's approach to physical activity:

Consistency: Engage in regular, consistent physical activity. Whether it's daily walks, yoga, dancing, or any other form of exercise, consistency is key.

Variety: Incorporate a variety of physical activities to keep things interesting and prevent boredom. This can include both aerobic (cardio) and strength-building exercises.

Moderation: Exercise should be enjoyable and sustainable. Avoid excessive or strenuous workouts that could lead to burnout or injury.

Mindful Movement: Approach exercise with mindfulness. Pay attention to your body's signals and adjust your activities accordingly.

Stress Reduction: Recognize the stress-reducing benefits of physical activity. Engaging in exercise can be a natural way to manage stress, which, in turn, can positively impact blood sugar levels.

Getting Started with Physical Activity

If you're new to regular physical activity or looking to rekindle your exercise routine, here are some steps to help you get started:

Consultation: If you have underlying health conditions or haven't been physically active for some time, consult with a healthcare provider before starting a new exercise regimen.

Set Realistic Goals: Define achievable fitness goals that align with your current fitness level and lifestyle.

Choose Enjoyable Activities: Select activities you genuinely enjoy. Whether it's dancing, hiking, swimming, or gardening, make exercise a pleasurable part of your routine.

Start Slowly: Begin at a pace that feels comfortable and gradually increase the duration and intensity of your workouts.

Stay Hydrated: Drink plenty of water before, during, and after exercise to stay properly hydrated.

Dr. Sebi's holistic approach to blood sugar control acknowledges the vital role of physical activity in achieving and maintaining stable blood sugar levels. As we continue our journey through this book, we'll delve deeper into other aspects of Dr. Sebi's philosophy, including the importance of sleep, stress reduction, hydration, and detoxification for holistic well-being.

<u>Chapter 7: The Healing Power of Sleep</u>

In our ongoing exploration of Dr. Sebi's holistic approach to blood sugar control, we arrive at a topic that is often overlooked but holds immense significance: the profound impact of sleep on blood sugar regulation and overall well-being.

Dr. Sebi's Perspective on Quality Sleep

Dr. Sebi recognized the vital role of sleep in achieving and maintaining optimal health. He believed that restful, restorative sleep was a cornerstone of his holistic approach to blood sugar control. Here's why quality sleep matters in Dr. Sebi's philosophy:

<u>Blood Sugar Regulation</u>: Sleep plays a crucial role in regulating blood sugar levels. During deep sleep, the body can balance hormones related to glucose metabolism.

<u>Cellular Repair</u>: Sleep is a time for cellular repair and rejuvenation. This includes repairing tissues and systems involved in blood sugar control.

<u>Stress Reduction</u>: A good night's sleep reduces stress levels, which can positively impact blood sugar regulation. Chronic stress is known to elevate blood sugar levels.

<u>Appetite and Hormones</u>: Sleep deprivation can disrupt hunger-regulating hormones, potentially leading to overeating and blood sugar spikes.

Creating Healthy Sleep Habits

Dr. Sebi's holistic approach to blood sugar control encourages the development of healthy sleep habits. Here are some key principles to consider:

<u>Consistent Sleep Schedule</u>: Go to bed and wake up at the same times each day, even on weekends. Consistency helps regulate your body's internal clock.

<u>Bedtime Routine Create a Relaxing</u>: Establish a calming routine before sleep, which can include activities like reading, meditation, or gentle stretching.

<u>Optimize Sleep Environment</u>: Ensure your sleep environment is conducive to rest. This includes a comfortable mattress and pillows, as well as a cool, dark, and quiet room.

<u>Limit Screen Time</u>: Reduce exposure to screens, such as phones and computers, at least an hour before bedtime. The blue light emitted from screens can disrupt sleep.

<u>Moderate Food and Fluids</u>: Avoid heavy meals, caffeine, and large quantities of fluids close to bedtime to prevent sleep disturbances.

<u>Physical Activity</u>: Engage in regular physical activity, but avoid vigorous exercise close to bedtime.

<u>Mindfulness and Relaxation</u>: Practice relaxation techniques, such as deep breathing or progressive muscle relaxation, to ease into a restful sleep.

Prioritizing Sleep for Blood Sugar Control

To support your blood sugar control journey, prioritize sleep as an integral part of your holistic approach:

Set a Sleep Goal: Aim for *7-9 hours* of quality sleep per night. Adjust your bedtime to achieve this goal.

Monitor Sleep Quality: Pay attention to the quality of your sleep. If you consistently wake up feeling unrested or experience sleep disturbances, consult with a healthcare provider.

Track Blood Sugar: If you have blood sugar concerns, consider tracking your levels to assess how sleep patterns may affect them.

Seek Professional Help: If you struggle with sleep disorders or chronic insomnia, consult with a sleep specialist or healthcare provider for guidance and solutions.

Dr. Sebi's holistic philosophy acknowledges that sleep is a natural, essential aspect of our lives, influencing not only blood sugar control but also overall well-being. As we continue our journey through this book, we'll delve into other facets of Dr. Sebi's approach, including stress reduction, hydration, detoxification, and the practical steps to implement his holistic principles for sustained blood sugar balance and vibrant health.

Chapter 8: Stress Reduction: Balancing Mind and Body

In our continued exploration of Dr. Sebi's holistic approach to blood sugar control, we encounter a critical aspect of his philosophy: the profound impact of stress on blood sugar levels and overall well-being. Dr. Sebi emphasized the importance of stress reduction as a key component of his holistic approach.

Dr. Sebi's Perspective on Stress

Dr. Sebi recognized that chronic stress could wreak havoc on the body's delicate balance, including blood sugar regulation. Stress triggers the release of hormones like cortisol and adrenaline, which can lead to elevated blood sugar levels. Here's why stress reduction matters in Dr. Sebi's philosophy:

Hormonal Balance: Chronic stress disrupts the balance of hormones involved in glucose metabolism, potentially leading to insulin resistance and blood sugar spikes.

Emotional Eating: Stress often triggers emotional eating, leading to the consumption of sugary or unhealthy foods that can negatively impact blood sugar.

Inflammation: Stress contributes to chronic inflammation, a factor in various health issues, including blood sugar imbalances.

Sleep Disruption: Stress can disrupt sleep patterns, affecting the body's ability to regulate blood sugar during restorative sleep.

Holistic Approaches to Stress Reduction

Dr. Sebi's holistic philosophy encourages stress reduction through a combination of mind-body practices and lifestyle choices. Here are some key principles to consider:

Mindfulness Meditation: Practice mindfulness meditation to cultivate awareness and reduce stress. This involves focusing on the present moment without judgment.

Yoga: Yoga combines physical postures, breathing exercises, and meditation to reduce stress and promote relaxation.

Deep Breathing: Engage in deep breathing exercises to activate the body's relaxation response. Techniques like diaphragmatic breathing can be particularly effective.

Nature Connection: Spending time in nature can have a calming effect on the mind and body. Nature walks or gardening are excellent stress-reducing activities.

Limiting Stimulants: Reduce or eliminate stimulants like caffeine and nicotine, which can exacerbate stress.

Time Management: Prioritize tasks and manage your time effectively to reduce the pressure of tight schedules.

Supportive Relationships: Cultivate supportive relationships with friends and family. Social connections are crucial for emotional well-being.

Incorporating Stress Reduction into Your Daily Life

To support your blood sugar control journey, consider integrating stress reduction practices into your daily routine:

Mindful Moments: Take short breaks throughout the day to practice mindfulness. Even a few minutes of deep breathing or mindful awareness can help reduce stress.

Physical Activity: Regular physical activity, such as walking or yoga, can help release tension and promote relaxation.

Journaling: Expressing your thoughts and emotions through journaling can be a therapeutic way to manage stress.

Hydration: Stay well-hydrated, as dehydration can exacerbate stress. Drink plenty of water throughout the day.

Herbal Support: Explore the use of herbal remedies, such as chamomile or lavender, known for their calming properties.

Stress reduction is an integral component of Dr. Sebi's holistic approach to blood sugar control and overall well-being. As we continue our journey through this book, we'll explore other facets of Dr. Sebi's philosophy, including hydration, detoxification, and practical steps to implement his holistic principles for sustained blood sugar balance and vibrant health.

Chapter 9: Hydration: The Elixir of Life

As we continue to explore Dr. Sebi's holistic approach to blood sugar control, we encounter a fundamental aspect of his philosophy: the significance of proper hydration for overall well-being and stable blood sugar levels.

Dr. Sebi's Perspective on Hydration

Dr. Sebi recognized that hydration is a cornerstone of health. He believed that maintaining proper fluid balance within the body was essential for efficient blood circulation, nutrient transport, and waste elimination. Here's why hydration matters in Dr. Sebi's philosophy:

Blood Sugar Regulation: Adequate hydration supports proper blood circulation, which is essential for the transportation of glucose and insulin throughout the body.

Toxin Removal: Hydration facilitates the removal of waste and toxins from the body, reducing the risk of inflammation and insulin resistance.

Digestive Health: Proper fluid balance aids in digestion, ensuring that nutrients are absorbed efficiently and blood sugar levels remain stable.

Appetite Control: Dehydration can sometimes be mistaken for hunger, leading to unnecessary snacking and potential blood sugar spikes.

Holistic Approaches to Hydration

Dr. Sebi's holistic philosophy encourages hydration through conscious fluid intake and the consumption of specific hydrating foods. Here are some key principles to consider:

Water Quality: Prioritize clean, purified water for hydration. Dr. Sebi emphasized the importance of avoiding tap water, which may contain impurities.

Herbal Infusions: Herbal teas, particularly those with hydrating herbs like chamomile or hibiscus, can be a flavorful and healthful way to increase fluid intake.

Hydrating Foods: Consume water-rich foods such as cucumbers, watermelon, and citrus fruits. These foods not only provide hydration but also essential nutrients.

Balanced Electrolytes: Dr. Sebi recommended natural electrolyte sources like coconut water to maintain electrolyte balance.

Limit Sugary Beverages: Avoid sugary and carbonated beverages, as they can disrupt blood sugar balance.

Incorporating Hydration into Your Daily Life

To support your blood sugar control journey and overall health, consider integrating these hydration practices into your daily routine:

Hydration Schedule: Develop a routine for drinking water throughout the day. Aim to consume water steadily rather than in large quantities all at once.

Herbal Hydration: Explore herbal infusions such as mint or ginger tea to increase fluid intake while enjoying added health benefits.

Fruit-Infused Water: Enhance the flavor of water by adding slices of fresh fruit, cucumber, or herbs like basil. This can make hydration more enjoyable.

Hydrating Snacks: Incorporate water-rich fruits and vegetables into your snacks. They can help satisfy hunger and support hydration.

Listen to Your Body: Pay attention to your body's signals for thirst. Sometimes, what may seem like hunger is actually a need for hydration.

The Gift of Hydration

Dr. Sebi's holistic approach recognizes that proper hydration is a foundational element of health and blood sugar control. As we continue our journey through this book, we'll explore the significance of detoxification, practical steps to implement Dr. Sebi's holistic principles, and the path to sustained blood sugar balance and vibrant well-being.

Chapter 10: Detoxification: Renewing Your Inner Terrain

In our final exploration of Dr. Sebi's holistic approach to blood sugar control, we encounter a transformative concept: detoxification. Dr. Sebi believed that regular detoxification was essential for clearing the body of accumulated waste, supporting optimal blood sugar levels, and fostering overall well-being.

Dr. Sebi's Perspective on Detoxification

Dr. Sebi viewed detoxification as a natural, rejuvenating process that allowed the body to heal and regain balance. He believed that toxins, waste, and mucus buildup in the body could disrupt blood sugar regulation. Here's why detoxification matters in Dr. Sebi's philosophy:

Cleansing the Blood: Detoxification helps cleanse the bloodstream of impurities, reducing the risk of inflammation and insulin resistance.

Cellular Renewal: It supports cellular regeneration, enabling cells involved in blood sugar regulation to function optimally.

Improved Digestion: Detoxification aids in better digestion and nutrient absorption, which are essential for stable blood sugar levels.

Weight Management: Eliminating waste and toxins can contribute to weight management, a critical factor in blood sugar control.

Holistic Approaches to Detoxification

Dr. Sebi's holistic philosophy encourages detoxification through dietary choices, fasting, herbal remedies, and lifestyle practices. Here are some key principles to consider:

Alkaline Diet: Prioritize an alkaline-rich diet, emphasizing fruits, vegetables, and herbs that support detoxification.

Herbal Detox: Incorporate detoxifying herbs such as dandelion, burdock root, and sarsaparilla into your dietary regimen.

Hydration: Proper hydration is essential for detoxification. Consume purified water and herbal teas to support the elimination of waste.

Fasting: Engage in periodic fasting or a fasting-mimicking diet to give your body a break and promote cleansing.

Colon Health: Dr. Sebi emphasized the importance of colon health. Colon-cleansing practices, such as enemas or colonics, were part of his approach.

Mindful Eating: Practice mindful eating to reduce overconsumption and promote healthy digestion.

Incorporating Detoxification into Your Life

To support your blood sugar control journey and overall well-being, consider integrating detoxification practices into your lifestyle:

Detox Schedule: Plan periodic detox periods, whether it's a weekend juice cleanse or a more extended fasting period. Consult with a healthcare provider before starting any detox regimen.

Herbal Support: Explore the use of detoxifying herbs as herbal infusions or supplements, following recommended dosages.

Colon Health: Consider colon-cleansing practices if you feel they are suitable for you. Consult with a healthcare provider or colon therapist for guidance.

Hydration: Stay well-hydrated during detoxification, as fluids are essential for flushing out toxins.

Mindful Detox: Approach detoxification with a mindful mindset. Listen to your body's signals and adjust your practices accordingly.

Embracing Holistic Well-Being

Dr. Sebi's holistic approach to blood sugar control acknowledges that detoxification is a natural and vital part of achieving and maintaining optimal health. By implementing the principles of detoxification alongside other holistic practices discussed in this book, you can embark on a path to sustained blood sugar balance, vibrant well-being, and a healthier, more balanced life.

As we conclude our journey through Dr. Sebi's holistic philosophy, remember that the holistic approach is not a one-size-fits-all solution. It's essential to consult with a healthcare provider or holistic practitioner who can guide you on the best practices and dietary choices tailored to your individual needs and circumstances.

Chapter 11: Practical Steps to Holistic Blood Sugar Control

In our final chapter, we bring together the essential principles of Dr. Sebi's holistic approach to blood sugar control and provide you with practical steps to implement these principles in your daily life. Achieving and maintaining stable blood sugar levels is a journey that requires commitment, awareness, and a holistic mindset.

Step 1: Embrace an Alkaline-Rich Diet

Prioritize fruits and vegetables that are high in alkaline minerals, such as leafy greens, kale, broccoli, and bell peppers.

Include herbs and spices like basil, oregano, and turmeric in your meals.

Choose plant-based proteins such as beans, lentils, and quinoa.

Limit or eliminate processed and sugary foods from your diet.

Step 2: Herbal Remedies for Blood Sugar Balance

Incorporate blood sugar-regulating herbs like bitter melon, burdock root, and cinnamon into your dietary regimen.

Consult with a healthcare provider or herbalist to determine the appropriate dosages and formulations for your needs.

Step 3: Practice Mindful Eating

Eat slowly and savor each bite, focusing on the flavors and textures of your food.

Pay attention to hunger and fullness cues to prevent overeating.

Be mindful of emotional eating triggers and find alternative ways to cope with stress or boredom.

Step 4: Engage in Regular Physical Activity

Establish a consistent exercise routine that includes both aerobic and strength-building exercises.

Aim for at least 150 minutes of moderate-intensity aerobic activity per week.

Incorporate movement into your daily life, such as walking or cycling.

Step 5: Prioritize Quality Sleep

Set a regular sleep schedule and aim for 7-9 hours of restful sleep per night.

Create a calming bedtime routine that includes relaxation techniques like deep breathing or meditation.

Step 6: Manage Stress Effectively

Practice stress reduction techniques such as mindfulness meditation, yoga, or deep breathing exercises.

Cultivate supportive relationships and seek emotional support when needed.

Step 7: Stay Hydrated

Consume purified water and herbal teas throughout the day to maintain proper hydration.

Enhance your hydration with water-rich foods like watermelon and cucumber.

Step 8: Periodic Detoxification

Plan periodic detox periods, such as a weekend juice cleanse or fasting-mimicking diet, to support your body's cleansing processes.

Consult with a healthcare provider before starting any detox regimen.

Step 9: Regular Monitoring

Monitor your blood sugar levels regularly, especially if you have diabetes or blood sugar concerns.

Keep a journal to track your progress and identify patterns related to diet, exercise, and lifestyle.

Step 10: Seek Professional Guidance

Consult with a healthcare provider, nutritionist, or holistic practitioner who can provide personalized guidance and support tailored to your unique needs and circumstances.

Consider regular check-ups to assess your overall health and blood sugar control.

Remember that achieving and maintaining stable blood sugar levels is a holistic endeavor that encompasses every aspect of your life. It's not a quick fix but a lifelong commitment to your well-being. By embracing these practical steps and incorporating Dr. Sebi's holistic principles into your daily routine, you can embark on a path to sustained blood sugar balance, vibrant health, and a more fulfilling life.

As we conclude this journey through Dr. Sebi's holistic philosophy, know that you have the knowledge and tools to make empowered choices for your health. Your journey towards optimal blood sugar control begins with the decision to prioritize your well-being and embrace a holistic approach to health and vitality.

<u>Chapter 12: The Journey Ahead: Holistic Blood Your Mastery Sugar</u>

As we conclude our journey through Dr. Sebi's holistic philosophy for blood sugar control, it's important to recognize that this journey is not a finite destination but an ongoing commitment to your well-being. Holistic blood sugar mastery is a lifelong path that requires dedication, self-awareness, and the willingness to make choices that support your health.

Embrace Your Holistic Lifestyle

The holistic approach to blood sugar control is not a quick fix but a comprehensive lifestyle that encompasses all aspects of your life. Embrace this lifestyle as a journey toward lasting well-being, vitality, and balanced blood sugar levels.

Ongoing Learning and Adaptation

Your health is a dynamic process, and your body's needs may change over time. Stay open to ongoing learning and adaptation. Be willing to explore new foods, exercise routines, and stress reduction techniques that align with your holistic journey.

The Power of Community and Support

Remember that you don't have to walk this path alone. Seek support from healthcare providers, holistic practitioners, and like-minded individuals who share your commitment to holistic health. Sharing your experiences and challenges can provide valuable insights and encouragement.

Celebrate Your Progress

Celebrate your achievements, no matter how small they may seem. Every positive step you take towards holistic blood sugar mastery is a victory. Recognize your efforts and the positive impact they have on your well-being.

The Holistic Approach to Life

As you continue your journey, apply the principles of holistic blood sugar control to all aspects of your life. Cultivate mindfulness, balance, and self-care in your relationships, work, and daily routines. The holistic approach extends beyond blood sugar—it's a philosophy for living your best, healthiest life.

Empower Yourself

You have the power to shape your health and future. Embrace this power and take charge of your well-being. Make informed choices, prioritize self-care, and remember that you are the steward of your body and mind.

Your Journey is Unique

Each person's journey to holistic blood sugar mastery is unique. What works for one individual may not be the same for another. Listen to your body, trust your intuition, and be patient with yourself as you navigate this path.

A Legacy of Health

By embracing the holistic principles of Dr. Sebi's philosophy, you are not only improving your own health but also contributing to a legacy of well-being for future generations. Your choices today have a lasting impact on your health and the health of those who follow in your footsteps.

Your Journey, Your Mastery

Holistic blood sugar mastery is a journey of self-discovery, empowerment, and vitality. It's a journey that allows you to take control of your health, find balance in your life, and embrace a future of well-being. As you continue your path, remember that you have the knowledge, tools, and inner strength to master your holistic blood sugar journey.

Thank you for embarking on this journey with us. Your commitment to holistic health is a powerful testament to your dedication to living a vibrant, balanced, and fulfilling life.

May your path be filled with vitality, joy, and lasting well-being.

Benefits of Reducing Blood Sugar Naturally and While You Sleep

The journey to reducing blood sugar naturally and fostering stable levels while you sleep is not merely a quest for numerical improvements on your glucose monitor. It's a profound journey toward overall well-being and vitality. Let's explore the benefits of achieving this harmony between natural blood sugar control and restful sleep.

1. Enhanced Energy Levels

Balanced blood sugar levels translate to consistent energy throughout the day. When your body efficiently regulates glucose, you experience fewer energy spikes and crashes. You'll find that you have sustained vitality for work, play, and all the activities you love.

2. Improved Mood and Mental Clarity

Blood sugar swings can affect your mood and mental clarity. Achieving natural blood sugar control can lead to a more stable emotional state and improved cognitive function. This translates to better focus, reduced brain fog, and a brighter outlook on life.

3. Weight Management

Maintaining stable blood sugar levels is closely linked to effective weight management. When your blood sugar is stable, you're less likely to experience intense hunger or cravings, making it easier to maintain a healthy weight or shed excess pounds.

4. Reduced Risk of Chronic Conditions

High blood sugar levels are associated with an increased risk of chronic conditions such as type 2 diabetes, heart disease, and metabolic syndrome. By reducing blood sugar naturally, you mitigate these risks and pave the way for a healthier, disease-free future.

5. Restorative Sleep

Quality sleep is essential for overall well-being, and it's intricately linked to blood sugar regulation. When your blood sugar levels remain steady during sleep, you experience more restorative rest. This means waking up refreshed, with improved memory consolidation and emotional balance.

6. Long-Term Health

The benefits of natural blood sugar control extend far into the future. By adopting holistic practices to reduce blood sugar, you're investing in your long-term health. You're nurturing a lifestyle that supports vitality, longevity, and an active, fulfilling life.

7. Reduced Risk of Complications

For those with diabetes, blood sugar control is crucial in preventing complications such as neuropathy, retinopathy, and kidney disease. Managing blood sugar naturally and through quality sleep reduces the risk of these debilitating complications.

8. Empowerment and Confidence

Taking charge of your blood sugar naturally and through sleep empowers you. It instills a sense of control over your health and well-being, fostering confidence in your ability to make informed choices for your body.

9. Vibrant Aging

Aging gracefully is a goal for many. By nurturing your blood sugar and sleep health, you promote vibrant aging. You can enjoy an active, fulfilling life well into your senior years, free from the burdens of age-related health concerns.

10. Improved Quality of Life

Ultimately, the benefits of reducing blood sugar naturally and while you sleep contribute to an improved overall quality of life. You experience greater physical vitality, emotional well-being, and the freedom to engage in the activities you love without being held back by blood sugar concerns.

As you embark on your journey to reduce blood sugar naturally and enjoy restorative sleep, keep these benefits in mind. They are the rewards of your commitment to holistic health and well-being.

Each step you take brings you closer to a life filled with vitality, joy, and lasting wellness.

1. Sugar-Free Strawberry Splash

- *Ingredients:*

    - 1 cup of fresh strawberries

    - 1/2 cucumber, peeled and chopped

    - 1/2 lime, juiced

    - 1 tablespoon of chia seeds

    - 1 cup of coconut water

- *Portion Measurements:* 1 serving (approx. 16 oz)

- *Nutritional Information (per serving):*

    - Calories: 120

    - Carbohydrates: 25g

    - Fiber: 8g

    - Protein: 3g

    - Fat: 3g

- *Prep Time:* 5 minutes

- *Instructions:*

1. Combine fresh strawberries, cucumber, lime juice, chia seeds, and coconut water in a blender.

2. Blend until sugar-free and strawberry-splendid.

3. Serve in a glass and enjoy this guilt-free strawberry splash!

2. Cinnamon Spice Sugar Soother

- *Ingredients:*

    - 1/2 cup of sweet potato, cooked and mashed

    - 1/2 teaspoon of cinnamon powder

    - 1/4 teaspoon of nutmeg powder

    - 1/2 teaspoon of vanilla extract

    - 1 cup of unsweetened almond milk

- *Portion Measurements:* 1 serving (approx. 16 oz)

- *Nutritional Information (per serving):*

    - Calories: 110

    - Carbohydrates: 24g

    - Fiber: 4g

    - Protein: 2g

    - Fat: 2g

- *Prep Time:* 10 minutes (to cook sweet potato)

- *Instructions:*

1. Blend mashed sweet potato, cinnamon powder, nutmeg powder, vanilla extract, and almond milk in a blender.

2. Blend until sugar-soothing and spiced to perfection.

3. Serve in a glass and savor the cinnamon spice soother!

<u>**3. Green Glucose Guardian**</u>

- *Ingredients:*

    - 2 cups of spinach

    - 1/2 cucumber, peeled and chopped

    - 1/2 green apple, cored and chopped

    - 1/2 lemon, juiced

    - 1 teaspoon of spirulina powder

    - 1 cup of filtered water

- *Portion Measurements:* 1 serving (approx. 16 oz)

- *Nutritional Information (per serving):*

    - Calories: 80

    - Carbohydrates: 18g

    - Fiber: 5g

    - Protein: 3g

    - Fat: 1g

- *Prep Time:* 5 minutes

- *Instructions:*

1. Combine spinach, cucumber, green apple, lemon juice, spirulina powder, and filtered water in a blender.

2. Blend until a green guardian for your glucose levels.

3. Serve in a glass and embrace the green glucose guardian!

4. Sweet Papaya Paradise

- *Ingredients:*
    - 1 cup of fresh papaya chunks
    - 1/2 cup of mango chunks
    - 1/2 lime, juiced
    - 1 tablespoon of flaxseed meal
    - 1 cup of coconut water
- *Portion Measurements:* 1 serving (approx. 16 oz)
- *Nutritional Information (per serving):*
    - Calories: 220
    - Carbohydrates: 48g
    - Fiber: 9g
    - Protein: 6g
    - Fat: 5g
- *Prep Time:* 5 minutes
- *Instructions:*

1. Blend fresh papaya chunks, mango chunks, lime juice, flaxseed meal, and coconut water in a blender.
2. Blend until a sweet paradise for your taste buds and blood sugar.
3. Serve in a glass and enjoy the sweet papaya paradise!

5. Vanilla Almond Bliss

- *Ingredients:*

    - 1 cup of unsweetened almond milk

    - 1/2 teaspoon of vanilla extract

    - 1/2 teaspoon of cinnamon powder

    - 1/4 teaspoon of nutmeg powder

    - 1/2 banana

- *Portion Measurements:* 1 serving (approx. 16 oz)

- *Nutritional Information (per serving):*

    - Calories: 90

    - Carbohydrates: 16g

    - Fiber: 3g

    - Protein: 2g

    - Fat: 2g

- *Prep Time:* 5 minutes

- *Instructions:*

1. Blend unsweetened almond milk, vanilla extract, cinnamon powder, nutmeg powder, and banana in a blender.

2. Blend until blissfully sugar-free and vanilla-kissed.

3. Serve in a glass and indulge in vanilla almond bliss!

<u>**6. Berry Balance Booster**</u>

- *Ingredients:*

    - <u>1 cup of mixed berries (strawberries, blueberries, raspberries)</u>

    - <u>1/2 cup of kale, stems removed</u>

    - <u>1 tablespoon of chia seeds</u>

    - <u>1/2 lemon, juiced</u>

    - <u>1 cup of coconut water</u>

- *Portion Measurements:* 1 serving (approx. 16 oz)

- *Nutritional Information (per serving):*

    - <u>Calories: 110</u>

    - <u>Carbohydrates: 24g</u>

    - <u>Fiber: 8g</u>

    - <u>Protein: 3g</u>

    - <u>Fat: 3g</u>

- *Prep Time:* 5 minutes

- *Instructions:*

1. <u>Combine mixed berries, kale, chia seeds, lemon juice, and coconut water in a blender.</u>

2. <u>Blend until a berry balance booster for your blood sugar.</u>

3. <u>Serve in a glass and boost your balance with berries!</u>

<u>**7. Mango Maple Morning Fuel**</u>

- *<u>Ingredients:</u>*

    - <u>1 cup of fresh mango chunks</u>

    - <u>1/2 banana</u>

    - <u>1 teaspoon of Dr. Sebi-approved sweetener (e.g., maple syrup)</u>

    - <u>1/2 lime, juiced</u>

    - <u>1 cup of coconut water</u>

- *<u>Portion Measurements:</u>* 1 serving (approx. 16 oz)

- *<u>Nutritional Information (per serving):</u>*

    - <u>Calories: 180</u>

    - <u>Carbohydrates: 42g</u>

    - <u>Fiber: 5g</u>

    - <u>Protein: 3g</u>

    - <u>Fat: 1g</u>

- *<u>Prep Time:</u>* 5 minutes

- *<u>Instructions:</u>*

1. <u>Blend fresh mango chunks, banana, maple syrup, lime juice, and coconut water in a blender.</u>

2. <u>Blend until morning fuel for your blood sugar and a sweet start to your day.</u>

3. <u>Serve in a glass and fuel your morning with mango maple goodness!</u>

8. Lemon Lime Zest Energizer

- *Ingredients:*
    - 1/2 lemon, juiced
    - 1/2 lime, juiced
    - 1/2 cucumber, peeled and chopped
    - 1/2 teaspoon of ginger powder
    - 1 cup of filtered water
- *Portion Measurements:* 1 serving (approx. 16 oz)
- *Nutritional Information (per serving):*
    - Calories: 15
    - Carbohydrates: 4g
    - Fiber: 1g
    - Protein: 1g
    - Fat: 0g
- *Prep Time:* 5 minutes
- *Instructions:*

1. Blend lemon juice, lime juice, cucumber, ginger powder, and filtered water in a blender.
2. Blend until an energizing zest for your day and blood sugar.
3. Serve in a glass and energize with lemon-lime zest!

9. Green Tea Glucose Guardian

- *Ingredients:*
    - 1 cup of brewed green tea, cooled
    - 1/2 cucumber, peeled and chopped
    - 1/2 teaspoon of matcha green tea powder
    - 1/2 lime, juiced
    - 1 teaspoon of chia seeds
- *Portion Measurements:* 1 serving (approx. 16 oz)
- *Nutritional Information (per serving):*
    - Calories: 10
    - Carbohydrates: 3g
    - Fiber: 2g
    - Protein: 1g
    - Fat: 1g
- *Prep Time:* 5 minutes (to brew and cool green tea)
- *Instructions:*

1. Blend brewed and cooled green tea, cucumber, matcha green tea powder, lime juice, and chia seeds in a blender.
2. Blend until a guardian for your glucose levels and green tea goodness.
3. Serve in a glass and protect your glucose with the green tea guardian!

10. Avocado Chocolate Delight

- *Ingredients:*

    - 1/2 avocado

    - 1 tablespoon of raw cacao powder

    - 1 teaspoon of Dr. Sebi-approved sweetener (e.g., agave nectar)

    - 1/2 teaspoon of vanilla extract

    - 1 cup of unsweetened almond milk

- *Portion Measurements:* 1 serving (approx. 16 oz)

- *Nutritional Information (per serving):*

    - Calories: 150

    - Carbohydrates: 11g

    - Fiber: 5g

    - Protein: 3g

    - Fat: 12g

- *Prep Time:* 5 minutes

- *Instructions:*

1. Blend avocado, raw cacao powder, sweetener, vanilla extract, and almond milk in a blender.

2. Blend until a delightful chocolate treat for your blood sugar.

3. Serve in a glass and relish the avocado chocolate delight!

These delightful and blood sugar-friendly smoothie recipes are aligned with Dr. Sebi's herbal alkaline diet principles. Enjoy them as part of a balanced diet, and consult with a healthcare professional or registered dietitian if you have specific dietary concerns or medical conditions.

Smoothie Benefits

1. Sugar-Free Strawberry Splash

- Benefits: Strawberries are low in sugar and high in fiber, which can help stabilize blood sugar levels. Cucumber adds hydration and aids in maintaining proper blood sugar balance.

2. Cinnamon Spice Sugar Soother

- Benefits: Cinnamon has been shown to improve insulin sensitivity and lower blood sugar levels. Sweet potato provides complex carbohydrates, contributing to steady glucose levels.

3. Green Glucose Guardian

- Benefits: Green apples are low in sugar and rich in fiber, promoting stable blood sugar. Spinach provides essential nutrients and antioxidants, supporting overall health.

4. Sweet Papaya Paradise

- Benefits: Papaya contains enzymes that may help improve digestion and regulate blood sugar. Mango adds natural sweetness and vitamins.

5. Vanilla Almond Bliss

- Benefits: Unsweetened almond milk is a low-carb alternative to regular milk, and cinnamon helps regulate blood sugar levels. Bananas provide potassium and natural sweetness.

6. Berry Balance Booster

- Benefits: Berries are low in sugar and packed with antioxidants, aiding in blood sugar control. Kale adds fiber and nutrients without raising blood sugar levels significantly.

7. Mango Maple Morning Fuel

- Benefits: Mangoes are rich in vitamins and minerals, and maple syrup is a natural sweetener with a lower glycemic index than refined sugar. Lime provides a refreshing twist.

8. Lemon Lime Zest Energizer

- Benefits: Lemons and limes are low in sugar and high in vitamin C, supporting blood sugar management. Cucumber adds hydration.

9. Green Tea Glucose Guardian

- Benefits: Green tea has been associated with improved insulin sensitivity and lower blood sugar levels. Matcha green tea powder provides antioxidants and a unique flavor.

10. Avocado Chocolate Delight

- Benefits: Avocado offers healthy fats and fiber, which can help stabilize blood sugar levels. Raw cacao is low in sugar and provides antioxidants, offering a chocolatey treat without the sugar spike.

These smoothies are designed to include ingredients that may aid in blood sugar regulation and diabetes management. However, it's crucial to consult with a healthcare professional or a registered dietitian for personalized dietary recommendations, especially if you have specific medical conditions or concerns regarding blood sugar.

Recipes

(These recipes incorporate whole grains, lean proteins, and plenty of vegetables, making them both nutritious and budget-friendly options for maintaining stable blood sugar levels. Enjoy experimenting with these delicious and wallet-friendly meals!)

Breakfast Recipes

<u>**Recipe 1: Oatmeal with Berries**</u>

Ingredients:

- 1/2 cup rolled oats
- 1 cup water or almond milk
- 1/2 cup mixed berries (strawberries, blueberries, raspberries)
- 1/4 teaspoon ground cinnamon
- 1 teaspoon honey (optional)
- Fresh mint leaves for garnish (optional)

Prep Time: 5 minutes Cook Time: 5 minutes Total Time: 10 minutes

Nutritional Information (Approximate):

- Calories: 250 kcal
- Fiber: 7g
- Protein: 5g

Instructions:

Prepare the Oats:

- In a small saucepan, bring 1 cup of water or almond milk to a gentle boil.

Add the Oats:

- Stir in 1/2 cup of rolled oats and reduce the heat to low.

Simmer:

- Let the oats simmer for about 5 minutes, stirring occasionally. Cook until they reach your desired consistency. If the mixture becomes too thick, you can add a bit more water or almond milk.

Add Cinnamon:

- Sprinkle 1/4 teaspoon of ground cinnamon into the oats and stir well. Cinnamon adds flavor and has potential blood sugar-regulating benefits.

Serve with Berries:

- Transfer the cooked oats to a bowl and top them with 1/2 cup of mixed berries. Berries are rich in antioxidants and add natural sweetness to your oatmeal.

Sweeten (Optional):

- If desired, drizzle 1 teaspoon of honey over the oatmeal for extra sweetness. Adjust the amount to your taste.
- Enjoy your delicious and nutritious oatmeal with berries is ready to enjoy! It's a hearty and wholesome breakfast that provides complex carbohydrates, fiber, and antioxidants to start your day right.

<u>**Recipe 2: Greek Yogurt Parfait**</u>

Ingredients:

- 1 cup Greek yogurt
- 1 ripe banana, sliced
- 2 tablespoons chopped nuts (e.g., almonds, walnuts)
- 1 tablespoon pure maple syrup (optional)

Prep Time: 5 minutes Total Time: 5 minutes

Nutritional Information (Approximate):

- Calories: 350 kcal
- Fiber: 4g
- Protein: 15g

Instructions:

Layer Ingredients:

- In a glass or bowl, layer Greek yogurt, sliced banana, and chopped nuts.

Sweeten (Optional):

- Drizzle 1 tablespoon of pure maple syrup over the parfait if desired.

Enjoy:

- Your creamy and satisfying Greek yogurt parfait is ready to enjoy. It's a protein-packed breakfast with natural sweetness and healthy fats.

Recipe 3: Avocado Toast

Ingredients:

- 2 slices of whole-grain bread
- 1 ripe avocado
- 2 poached or fried eggs
- Pinch of black pepper
- Pinch of salt

Prep Time: 10 minutes Cook Time: 5 minutes Total Time: 15 minutes

Nutritional Information (Approximate):

- Calories: 350 kcal
- Fiber: 10g
- Protein: 14g

Instructions:

Toast the Bread:

- Toast two slices of whole-grain bread to your desired level of crispiness.

Prepare Avocado:

- While the bread is toasting, cut the ripe avocado in half, remove the pit, and scoop out the flesh.

Mash Avocado:

- Mash the avocado with a fork until it reaches a creamy consistency.

Prepare Eggs:

- Poach or fry two eggs in a non-stick skillet to your preferred level of doneness.

Assemble:

- Spread the mashed avocado evenly on the toasted bread slices.
- Place one poached or fried egg on each slice.
- Season with a pinch of black pepper and salt.

Enjoy:

- Your nutritious and savory avocado toast is ready to enjoy. It's a satisfying breakfast rich in healthy fats and protein.

<u>**Recipe 4: Chia Seed Pudding**</u>

Ingredients:

- 2 tablespoons chia seeds
- 1 cup unsweetened almond milk
- 1/2 teaspoon pure vanilla extract
- Fresh berries for topping

Prep Time: 5 minutes (plus overnight soaking) Total Time: 5 minutes prep + overnight soaking

Nutritional Information (Approximate):

- Calories: 180 kcal
- Fiber: 10g
- Protein: 4g

Instructions:

Mix Ingredients:

- In a bowl, combine chia seeds, almond milk, and vanilla extract. Stir well.

Soak Overnight:

- Cover the bowl and refrigerate overnight (or for at least 4 hours) to allow the chia seeds to absorb the liquid and create a pudding-like consistency.

Top with Berries:

- Before serving, top your chia seed pudding with fresh berries.

Enjoy:

- Your creamy and nutritious chia seed pudding is ready to enjoy. It's a great make-ahead breakfast option rich in fiber and omega-3 fatty acids.

<u>**Recipe 5: Veggie Scramble**</u>

Ingredients:

- 2 large eggs
- 1/2 cup bell peppers (any color), diced
- 1/4 cup onions, diced
- 1/2 cup spinach, chopped
- Salt and pepper to taste
- Cooking oil (e.g., olive oil or cooking spray)

Prep Time: 5 minutes Cook Time: 10 minutes Total Time: 15 minutes

Nutritional Information (Approximate):

- Calories: 250 kcal
- Fiber: 3g
- Protein: 14g

Instructions:

Sauté Vegetables:

- Heat a non-stick skillet over medium heat. Add a small amount of cooking oil or use cooking spray.
- Sauté diced bell peppers and onions until they become tender.

Add Spinach:

- Add chopped spinach to the skillet and continue cooking until it wilts.

Scramble Eggs:

- In a bowl, beat the eggs with a pinch of salt and pepper.
- Pour the beaten eggs into the skillet with the sautéed vegetables.

Cook and Stir:

- Stir gently as the eggs cook, ensuring they mix well with the vegetables.

Serve:

- When the eggs are fully cooked and no longer runny, transfer the veggie scramble to a plate.

Enjoy:

- Your flavorful and protein-rich veggie scramble is ready to enjoy. It's a savory and filling breakfast.

<u>**Recipe 6: Whole-Grain Pancakes**</u>

Ingredients:

- 1 cup whole-grain flour
- 1 tablespoon baking powder
- 1/4 teaspoon salt
- 1 cup unsweetened almond milk
- 1 large egg
- 1 tablespoon honey (optional)
- Cooking oil (e.g., olive oil or cooking spray)

Prep Time: 10 minutes Cook Time: 15 minutes Total Time: 25 minutes

Nutritional Information (Approximate):

- Calories: 280 kcal per serving (3 pancakes)
- Fiber: 4g
- Protein: 7g per serving (3 pancakes)

Instructions:

Mix Dry Ingredients:

- In a bowl, whisk together whole-grain flour, baking powder, and salt.

Combine Wet Ingredients:

- In a separate bowl, whisk together almond milk, egg, and honey (if using).

Combine Mixtures:

- Pour the wet ingredients into the dry ingredients and stir until just combined. Do not overmix; it's okay if there are lumps.

Heat Skillet:

- Heat a non-stick skillet over medium heat. Add a small amount of cooking oil or use cooking spray to prevent sticking.

Cook Pancakes:

- Pour 1/4 cup of pancake batter onto the skillet for each pancake. Cook until bubbles form on the surface, then flip and cook until golden brown on both sides.

Serve:

- Stack your whole-grain pancakes on a plate.
- Enjoy your wholesome and hearty whole-grain pancakes with some fresh fruit.

<u>**Recipe 7: Smoothie Bowl**</u>

Ingredients (Approximately 2 servings):

- 2 ripe bananas
- 1 cup frozen mixed berries (strawberries, blueberries, raspberries)
- 1/2 cup Greek yogurt
- 1/2 cup almond milk (or your choice of milk)
- 2 tablespoons honey or maple syrup (optional, for sweetness)
- Toppings: Sliced bananas, fresh berries, granola, chia seeds, shredded coconut, and a drizzle of honey (customize to your liking)

Prep Time: 5 minutes Cook Time: 0 minutes (no cooking required) Total Time: 5 minutes

Nutritional Information (Approximate):

- Calories: Approximately 350 kcal
- Fiber: Approximately 10g
- Protein:

Instructions:

Prepare the Smoothie Base:

- In a blender, combine the ripe bananas, frozen mixed berries, Greek yogurt, almond milk, and honey or maple syrup (if desired).
- Blend until you achieve a smooth and creamy consistency.

Assemble the Bowl:

- Pour the smoothie into serving bowls.
- Top it with your choice of sliced bananas, fresh berries, granola, chia seeds, shredded coconut, and a drizzle of honey.

Enjoy:

- Grab a spoon and dive into your delicious and nutritious smoothie bowl. Feel free to customize the toppings based on your preferences.

<u>**Recipe 8: Breakfast Burrito**</u>

Ingredients (Approximately 2 servings):

- 4 large eggs
- Salt and pepper to taste
- 2 large whole-grain or spinach tortillas
- 1/2 cup black beans, drained and rinsed
- 1/2 cup diced bell peppers (any color)
- 1/2 cup diced onions
- 1/2 cup diced tomatoes
- 1/4 cup shredded cheddar cheese
- Salsa, avocado slices, and fresh cilantro for garnish (optional)

Prep Time: 10 minutes Cook Time: 10 minutes Total Time: 20 minutes

Nutritional Information (Approximate):

- Calories: 360 kcal per serving
- Fiber: 5g per serving
- Protein: 14g per serving

Instructions:

Scramble the Eggs:

- In a bowl, whisk the eggs until well beaten.
- Heat a non-stick skillet over medium heat, add a touch of cooking oil or cooking spray.
- Pour the beaten eggs into the skillet and season with salt and pepper.
- Gently scramble the eggs until they are fully cooked but still moist. Remove from heat.

Assemble the Burrito:

- Lay out the tortillas on a clean, flat surface.
- Divide the scrambled eggs evenly between the two tortillas.

Add the Fillings:

- Add black beans, diced bell peppers, diced onions, diced tomatoes, and shredded cheddar cheese on top of the scrambled eggs.

Roll the Burritos:

- Fold in the sides of each tortilla.
- Roll up the tortilla from the bottom to enclose the fillings and create a burrito.

Serve:

- You can serve the breakfast burritos whole or slice them in half for easier handling.
- Garnish with salsa, avocado slices, and fresh cilantro if desired.

<u>**Recipe 9: Fruit Salad**</u>

Ingredients:

- Assorted seasonal fruits (e.g., apples, pears, grapes)
- 1 tablespoon Fresh lemon juice
- Ground cinnamon

Prep Time: 10 minutes Total Time: 10 minutes

Nutritional Information (Approximate):

- Calories: Varies based on fruit selection
- Fiber: Varies based on fruit selection
- Protein: Varies based on fruit selection

Instructions:

Prepare Fruits:

- Wash and chop the seasonal fruits of your choice into bite-sized pieces. Apples and pears work well, and grapes add sweetness.

Drizzle Lemon Juice:

- Squeeze fresh lemon juice over the fruit to enhance the flavors and prevent browning.

Add a Pinch of Cinnamon:

- Sprinkle a pinch of ground cinnamon over the fruit for a delightful aroma and extra flavor.

Toss and Serve:

- Gently toss the fruit to coat them with lemon juice and cinnamon.

Enjoy:

- Your refreshing and naturally sweet fruit salad is ready to enjoy as a healthy dessert or side dish.

<u>**Recipe 10: Homemade Muesli**</u>

Ingredients:

- 1 cup Rolled oats
- 1/4 cup Chopped nuts such as almonds, walnuts, or pecans
- 1/4 cup Dried fruits such as raisins, cranberries, or apricots
- 2 tablespoons Honey or to taste
- 1/2 cup Yogurt for serving
- 1/2 cup Fresh berries for serving

Prep Time: 10 minutes Total Time: 10 minutes

Nutritional Information (Approximate):

- Calories: Varies based on portion size and ingredients
- Fiber: Varies based on portion size and ingredients
- Protein: Varies based on portion size and ingredients

Instructions:

Mix Dry Ingredients:

- In a bowl, combine rolled oats, chopped nuts, and dried fruits. You can adjust the quantities to your liking.

Drizzle Honey:

- Drizzle a touch of honey over the dry mixture to add sweetness and help bind the ingredients together.

Serve with Yogurt:

- Serve the muesli with a generous dollop of yogurt. Greek yogurt works well for added creaminess and protein.

Add Fresh Berries:

- Top the muesli with fresh berries of your choice, such as strawberries and blueberries.

Enjoy:

- Your homemade muesli with yogurt and fresh berries is ready to enjoy as a nutritious and satisfying dinner.

<u>Lunch Recipes</u>

<u>**Recipe 1: Quinoa Salad**</u>

Ingredients:

- 1 cup cooked quinoa

- 1/2 cup chickpeas

- 1/2 cup cucumber, diced

- 1/2 cup cherry tomatoes, halved

- 2 tablespoons lemon vinaigrette

- Salt and pepper to taste

Portions: This recipe makes approximately 2 servings.

Prep Time: 15 minutes Cook Time: N/A Total Time: 15 minutes

Nutritional Information (Approximate per serving):

- Calories: 250 kcal
- Fiber: 6g
- Protein: 8g

Instructions:

1. Prepare Quinoa Salad:

- In a bowl, combine 1 cup of cooked quinoa, 1/2 cup of chickpeas, 1/2 cup of diced cucumber, and 1/2 cup of halved cherry tomatoes.

- Drizzle 2 tablespoons of lemon vinaigrette over the mixture.

- Season with salt and pepper to taste.

<u>**Recipe 2: Vegetable Stir-Fry**</u>

Ingredients:

- 2 cups broccoli

- 1 cup bell peppers, sliced

- 1 cup snap peas

- 1 cup tofu or tempeh, cubed

- 3 tablespoons stir-fry sauce

- Salt and pepper to taste

Portions: This recipe makes approximately 2 servings.

Prep Time: 20 minutes Cook Time: 20 minutes Total Time: 40 minutes

Nutritional Information (Approximate per serving - without rice):

- Calories: 250 kcal
- Fiber: 5g
- Protein: 10g

Instructions:

1. Prepare Vegetable Stir-Fry:

   - In a pan, sauté 2 cups of broccoli, 1 cup of sliced bell peppers, 1 cup of snap peas, and 1 cup of tofu or tempeh.

   - Add 3 tablespoons of stir-fry sauce.

   - Season with salt and pepper to taste.

<u>**Recipe 3: Tuna Salad Wrap**</u>

Ingredients:

- 1 can of tuna in water, drained
- 2 tablespoons Greek yogurt
- 1/4 cup diced celery
- 1/4 teaspoon Dijon mustard
- Salt and pepper to taste
- Whole-grain tortillas
- Lettuce leaves
- Sliced tomatoes

Prep Time: 10 minutes Total Time: 10 minutes

Nutritional Information (Approximate):

- Calories: 280 kcal per wrap
- Fiber: 5g
- Protein: 25g per wrap

Instructions:

1. Prepare Tuna Salad:

   - In a bowl, mix drained tuna, Greek yogurt, diced celery, Dijon mustard, salt, and pepper. Combine until well blended.

2. Assemble Wraps:

   - Lay out whole-grain tortillas.

3. Place a lettuce leaf on each tortilla.

   - Spoon the tuna salad mixture onto the lettuce.

4. Add Tomatoes:

   - Top with sliced tomatoes.

5. Wrap:

   - Roll up the tortillas, folding in the sides as you go.

6. Enjoy:

   - Your tasty tuna salad wrap is ready to enjoy. It's a protein-packed and satisfying lunch.

<u>Recipe 4: Sweet Potato and Black Bean Bowl</u>

Ingredients:

- 1 medium sweet potato, peeled and cubed
- 1/2 cup canned black beans, drained and rinsed
- 1/2 cup corn kernels (frozen or canned)
- 1/2 avocado, diced
- Fresh lime juice
- Fresh cilantro leaves (optional)
- Lime wedges for garnish (optional)

Prep Time: 10 minutes Cook Time: 20 minutes Total Time: 30 minutes

Nutritional Information (Approximate):

- Calories: 320 kcal
- Fiber: 11g
- Protein: 7g

Instructions:

1. Roast Sweet Potato:

   - Preheat your oven to 400°F (200°C).

2. Toss sweet potato cubes with a drizzle of olive oil, salt, and pepper.

   - Roast for about 20 minutes or until they are tender and slightly crispy.

3. Assemble Bowl:

   - In a bowl, combine roasted sweet potato, black beans, and corn.

4. Add Avocado:

   - Top the mixture with diced avocado.

5. Squeeze Lime:

   - Squeeze fresh lime juice over the bowl for a burst of flavor.

6. Garnish (Optional):

   - If desired, garnish with fresh cilantro leaves and lime wedges.

7. Enjoy:

   - Your colorful and nutritious sweet potato and black bean bowl is ready to enjoy. It's a filling and balanced lunch option.

<u>**Recipe 5: Lemon Garlic Shrimp Scampi**</u>

Ingredients:

- 1 pound large shrimp, peeled and deveined
- 8 oz. linguine or spaghetti
- 3 tablespoons unsalted butter
- 3 cloves garlic, minced
- Zest and juice of 1 lemon
- 1/4 cup white wine (optional)
- 2 tablespoons fresh parsley, chopped
- Salt and freshly ground black pepper, to taste
- Red pepper flakes (optional, for some heat)
- Grated Parmesan cheese, for garnish

Portions: This recipe makes approximately 4 serving.

Nutritional Information (Approximate):

- Calories: 320 kcal per serving
- Protein: 24g
- Carbohydrates: 29g

Instructions:

1. Cook Pasta:
   - Cook the linguine or spaghetti according to the package instructions until al dente. Drain and set aside.
2. Sauté Shrimp:
   - In a large skillet, melt 2 tablespoons of butter over medium-high heat. Add the minced garlic and sauté for about 1 minute until fragrant.
3. Cook Shrimp:
   - Add the shrimp to the skillet in a single layer. Cook for about 2 minutes on each side until they turn pink and opaque. Remove the shrimp from the skillet and set them aside.
4. Prepare Scampi Sauce:
   - In the same skillet, add the remaining 1 tablespoon of butter, lemon zest, lemon juice, and white wine (if using). Cook for 2-3 minutes, allowing the sauce to reduce slightly.
5. Combine Pasta and Shrimp:
   - Return the cooked pasta to the skillet and toss it in the scampi sauce until well coated.
6. Add Shrimp and Season:
   - Add the cooked shrimp back to the skillet. Sprinkle with chopped fresh parsley and season with salt, black pepper, and red pepper flakes if you like it spicy.
7. Serve:
   - Divide the Lemon Garlic Shrimp Scampi among four plates. Garnish with grated Parmesan cheese if desired.
8. Enjoy:
   - Serve immediately while it's hot. This dish is bursting with flavor, thanks to the zesty lemon and garlic, and is sure to satisfy your taste buds.

Recipe 6: Hummus and Veggie Wrap

Ingredients:

- Hummus
- Whole-grain tortilla
- Sliced cucumbers
- Carrots
- Spinach
- Salt and pepper to taste

Portions: This recipe makes approximately 1 serving.

Prep Time: 10 minutes Cook Time: N/A Total Time: 10 minutes

Nutritional Information (Approximate per serving):

- Calories: 280 kcal
- Fiber: 7g
- Protein: 8g

Instructions:

- Assemble Hummus and Veggie Wrap:

- Spread hummus on a whole-grain tortilla.

- Add sliced cucumbers, carrots, and fresh spinach.

- Season with salt and pepper to taste.

<u>**Recipe 7: Brown Rice Bowl**</u>

Ingredients:

- 1 cup Cooked brown rice
- 1 cup Sautéed mushrooms
- 1 cup Fresh spinach
- 1 Large Fried egg
- 1-2 tablespoons of Soy sauce
- Salt and pepper to taste

Portions: This recipe makes approximately 1 serving.

Prep Time: 20 minutes Cook Time: 20 minutes Total Time: 40 minutes

Nutritional Information (Approximate per serving):

- Calories: 400 kcal
- Fiber: 6g
- Protein: 15g

Instructions:

- Prepare Brown Rice Bowl:

- Top cooked brown rice with sautéed mushrooms and fresh spinach.

- Add a perfectly fried egg on top.

- Drizzle with soy sauce, and season with salt and pepper to taste.

<u>**Recipe 8: Chickpea Salad**</u>

Ingredients:

- 1 can canned Chickpeas
- ¼ cup diced Red onion
- ¼ cup diced Bell pepper
- Handful, roughly chopped Fresh parsley
- 2-3 tablespoons Lemon-tahini dressing
- Salt and pepper to taste

Portions: This recipe makes approximately 2 servings.

Prep Time: 15 minutes Cook Time: N/A Total Time: 15 minutes

Nutritional Information (Approximate per serving):

- Calories: 250 kcal
- Fiber: 8g
- Protein: 7g

Instructions:

- Prepare Chickpea Salad:

- Mix canned chickpeas, diced red onion, diced bell pepper, fresh parsley, and drizzle with lemon-tahini dressing.

- Season with salt and pepper to taste.

<u>**Recipe 9: Peanut Butter and Banana Sandwich**</u>

Ingredients:

- Natural peanut butter
- Whole-grain bread
- Sliced banana
- Honey

Portions: This recipe makes approximately 1 serving.

Prep Time: 5 minutes Cook Time: N/A Total Time: 5 minutes

Nutritional Information (Approximate per serving):

- Calories: 350 kcal
- Fiber: 6g
- Protein: 9g

Instructions:

- Assemble Peanut Butter and Banana Sandwich:

- Spread natural peanut butter on whole-grain bread.

- Add sliced banana, and drizzle with honey.

<u>**Recipe 10: Vegetable Frittata**</u>

Ingredients (4 servings):

- 6 large eggs
- 1 1/2 cups diced zucchini
- 1/2 cup diced onions
- 1/2 cup crumbled feta cheese
- Salt and pepper to taste

Prep Time: 15 minutes Cook Time: 20 minutes Total Time: 35 minutes

Nutritional Information (Approximate per serving):

- Calories: 180 kcal
- Fiber: 2g
- Protein: 10g

Instructions:

- Prepare Vegetable Frittata:

- In an oven-safe skillet, sauté the diced zucchini and onions until they are tender and slightly caramelized. Season with salt and pepper to taste.

- Preheat your oven to 350°F (175°C).

- In a separate bowl, beat the eggs until well mixed.

- Pour the beaten eggs evenly over the sautéed vegetables in the skillet.

- Sprinkle crumbled feta cheese evenly over the mixture.

- Place the skillet in the preheated oven and bake until the frittata is set and slightly golden on top. This typically takes about 15-20 minutes, but times may vary, so keep an eye on it.

- Once done, remove the frittata from the oven and let it cool for a few minutes.

- Slice the frittata into wedges.

- Your flavorful and protein-packed vegetable frittata is ready to enjoy. It makes for a delicious lunch or brunch option.

<u>Dinner Recipes</u>

<u>Dinner Recipes</u>

Recipe 1: Pasta Primavera

Ingredients:

- Whole-grain pasta (4 cups)
- Mixed vegetables (2 cups)
- Tomato sauce (2 cups)
- Olive oil (2 tablespoons)
- Salt and pepper to taste

Prep Time: 15 minutes Portions: 4 servings

Nutritional Information (Per Serving):

- Calories: 450 kcal
- Fiber: 5g
- Protein: 12g

Instructions:

- Prepare Pasta Primavera:

- Cook whole-grain pasta according to package instructions until al dente. Drain and set aside.

- In a pan, heat olive oil over medium heat.

- Sauté mixed vegetables until tender-crisp.

- Toss the sautéed vegetables with tomato sauce.

- Serve the vegetable sauce over cooked pasta.

<u>**Recipe 2: Baked Sweet Potatoes**</u>

Ingredients:

- Sweet potatoes (4 medium-sized)
- Black beans (1 can)
- Salsa (1 cup)
- Greek yogurt (1/2 cup)

Prep Time: 10 minutes Portions: 4 servings

Nutritional Information (Per Serving):

- Calories: 350 kcal
- Fiber: 10g
- Protein: 10g

Instructions:

- Prepare Baked Sweet Potatoes:

- Preheat your oven to 375°F (190°C).

- Scrub sweet potatoes and prick them with a fork.

- Bake for about 45-50 minutes or until tender.

- Split each baked sweet potato open.

- Top with black beans or salsa.

<u>**Recipe 3: Vegetable Chili**</u>

Ingredients:

- Mixed vegetables (4 cups)
- Beans (2 cans)
- Tomatoes (1 can)
- Chili powder (2 tablespoons)
- Spices
- Brown rice (4 servings)

Prep Time: 20 minutes Portions: 4 servings

Nutritional Information (Per Serving):

- Calories: 400 kcal
- Fiber: 15g
- Protein: 10g

Instructions:

- Prepare Vegetable Chili:

- Sauté mixed vegetables until they start to soften.

- Add beans, diced tomatoes, chili powder, and your choice of spices.

- Simmer until flavors meld.

- Serve the vegetable chili over cooked brown rice.

Recipe 4: Stuffed Bell Peppers

Ingredients:

- Bell peppers (4)
- Quinoa (1 cup)
- Black beans (1 can)
- Corn (1 cup)
- Diced tomatoes (1 can)

Prep Time: 25 minutes Portions: 4 servings

Nutritional Information (Per Serving):

- Calories: 300 kcal
- Fiber: 10g
- Protein: 10g

Instructions:

- Prepare Stuffed Bell Peppers:

- Cut the tops off bell peppers and remove seeds and membranes.

- In a bowl, mix cooked quinoa, black beans, corn, and diced tomatoes.

- Fill each bell pepper with the quinoa and vegetable mixture.

- Bake until peppers are tender.

<u>**Recipe 5: Lentil Soup**</u>

Ingredients:

- Lentils (1 cup)
- Onions (1)
- Carrots (2)
- Celery (2 stalks)
- Vegetable broth (4 cups)
- Herbs and spices

Prep Time: 15 minutes Portions: 4 servings

Nutritional Information (Per Serving):

- Calories: 250 kcal
- Fiber: 12g
- Protein: 15g

Instructions:

- Prepare Lentil Soup

- Sauté onions, carrots, and celery until tender.

- Add lentils and vegetable broth.

- Season with herbs and spices.

- Simmer until lentils are cooked.

<u>**Recipe 6: Baked Salmon with Veggies**</u>

Ingredients:

- 4 Salmon fillets (4-6 ounces)
- 2 tablespoon of Lemon juice
- 2 pinches of fresh herbs
- 2 tablespoons of Olive oil
- 2 cups of Assorted roasted vegetables (e.g., broccoli, carrots, and bell peppers)

Prep Time: 20 minutes Portions: 4 servings

Nutritional Information (Per Serving):

- Calories: 350 kcal
- Fiber: 6g
- Protein: 30g

Instructions:

- Prepare Baked Salmon with Veggies

- Season salmon fillets with lemon juice and fresh herbs.

- Bake salmon with a medley of roasted vegetables until salmon flakes easily.

<u>**Recipe 7: Mushroom and Spinach Quesadillas**</u>

Ingredients:

- Mushrooms (2 cups)
- Spinach (2 cups)
- Whole-grain tortillas (4)
- Cheese (1 cup)
- Olive oil (2 tablespoons)

Prep Time: 15 minutes Portions: 4 servings

Nutritional Information (Per Serving):

- Calories: 350 kcal
- Fiber: 6g
- Protein: 15g

Instructions:

- Prepare Mushroom and Spinach Quesadillas:

- Sauté mushrooms and spinach until wilted.

- Place sautéed mushrooms and spinach between whole-grain tortillas with cheese.

- Cook until crispy.

<u>**Recipe 8: Cauliflower and Chickpea Curry**</u>

Ingredients:

- Cauliflower (1 head)
- Chickpeas (2 cans)
- Curry sauce (2 cups)
- Brown rice (4 servings)

Prep Time: 20 minutes Portions: 4 servings

Nutritional Information (Per Serving):

- Calories: 350 kcal
- Fiber: 10g
- Protein: 10g

Instructions:

- Prepare Cauliflower and Chickpea Curry

- Cook cauliflower and chickpeas in a fragrant curry sauce.

- Serve over cooked brown rice.

<u>**Recipe 9: Spaghetti Squash with Marinara**</u>

Ingredients:

- Spaghetti squash (2)
- Marinara sauce (2 cups)
- Grated Parmesan

Prep Time: 15 minutes Portions: 4 servings

Nutritional Information (Per Serving):

- Calories: 200 kcal
- Fiber: 8g
- Protein: 4g

Instructions:

- Prepare Spaghetti Squash with Marinara

- Roast spaghetti squash until tender.

- Top with homemade marinara sauce and grated Parmesan.

Recipe 10: Bean and Rice Burrito Bowl

Ingredients:

- Brown rice (4 servings)
- Black beans (2 cans)
- Onions and peppers (2 cups)
- Salsa (1 cup)
- Avocado (2)

Prep Time: 15 minutes Portions: 4 servings

Nutritional Information (Per Serving):

- Calories: 450 kcal
- Fiber: 12g
- Protein: 10g

Instructions:

- Prepare Bean and Rice Burrito Bowl

- Cook brown rice and black beans.

- Sauté onions and peppers.

- Layer cooked brown rice with black beans, sautéed onions, and peppers.

- Top with salsa and avocado.

<u>7 – Day Meal Plan</u>

(This is just one example of our 7-day meal plan. With 10 breakfast options, 10 lunch choices, and 10 dinner recipes, you can create an astonishing 1 quintillion unique 7-day meal plan combinations.)

<u>**Day 1:**</u>

Breakfast: Oatmeal with Berries

Lunch: Tuna Salad Wrap

Dinner: Vegetable Chili

<u>**Day 2:**</u>

Breakfast: Greek Yogurt Parfait

Lunch: Sweet Potato and Black Bean Bowl

Dinner: Stuffed Bell Peppers

<u>**Day 3:**</u>

Breakfast: Chia Seed Pudding

Lunch: Chickpea Salad

Dinner: Spaghetti Squash with Marinara

<u>**Day 4:**</u>

Breakfast: Avocado Toast

Lunch: Vegetable Stir-Fry

Dinner: Baked Salmon with Veggies

<u>**Day 5:**</u>

Breakfast: Whole-Grain Pancakes

Lunch: Lemon Garlic Shrimp Scampi

Dinner: Lentil Soup

<u>**Day 6:**</u>

Breakfast: Smoothie Bowl

Lunch: Quinoa Salad

Dinner: Bean and Rice Burrito Bowl

<u>**Day 7:**</u>

Breakfast: Fruit Salad

Lunch: Hummus and Veggie Wrap

Dinner: Mushroom and Spinach Quesadillas

(This meal plan provides a variety of balanced and nutritious meals, including a mix of whole grains, lean proteins, healthy fats, and plenty of vegetables and fruits. You can adjust portion sizes to meet your specific dietary needs and preferences.)

Don't forget to stay hydrated by drinking plenty of water throughout the day. Enjoy the journey!!!